COMPLETE GUIDE TO IRRITABLE BOWEL SYNDROME [IBS]

Comprehensive Strategies For Symptoms Relief, Effective Treatments, Proven Diet Plans, Natural Remedies, And Lifestyle Changes For Lasting Wellness

DEHART HAIRSTON

© [DEHART HAIRSTON], [2024]

All rights reserved. No part of this publication may be reproduced, distributed, or transmitted in any form or by any means, including photocopying, recording, or other electronic or mechanical methods, without the prior written permission of the publisher, except in the case of brief quotations embodied in critical reviews and certain other noncommercial uses permitted by copyright law.

DISCLAIMER

This book's content is only intended for general informative purposes. At the time of writing, the author has taken every precaution to guarantee that the material is correct and current. Nevertheless, the author disclaims all explicit and implicit representations and guarantees about the availability, appropriateness, correctness, completeness, and usefulness of the material on these pages.

Since the author is not a licensed medical practitioner, the material in this book shouldn't be interpreted as medical advice. Before making any modifications to their diet, exercise regimen, or medical treatment, readers are urged to speak with a licensed healthcare provider.

Moreover, the author has no connection to any of the businesses, organizations, or people that are discussed in this book. Any mentions of goods, services, businesses, or people are purely informative and do not indicate endorsement or suggestion.

This book's content is entirely dependent on the author's expertise, study, and comprehension of the topic. Despite having taken reasonable care to offer correct information, the author disclaims all liability for any mistakes or omissions in the material as well as for any losses, harm, or damages resulting from using the information.

It is recommended that readers use their own judgment and discretion when applying the knowledge in this book to their own situations. The use or implementation of any material in this book may result in unfavorable repercussions, directly or indirectly, for which the author assumes no liability.

By reading this book, you agree to release and hold the author harmless from any claims, losses, liabilities, costs, or expenditures resulting from or related to the use of the information you get from it.

Table of Contents

CHAPTER 1 15
Understanding Irritable Bowel Syndrome (Ibs).....15
What Is Ibs?...15
Symptoms Of Ibs 16
Types Of Ibs..17
1. IBS with Constipation (IBS-C): 17
2. IBS with diarrhea (IBS-D): 17
3. Mixed IBS (IBS-M):...18
Causes And Triggers..18
1. Stomach Dysfunction:..19
2. Dietary Factors:..19
3. Stress and Mental Health: 20
4. Gut Microbiota:...20

CHAPTER 2 23
Diagnosing Ibs 23
Criteria For Diagnosis 23
Medical History And Physical Examination...........24
Diagnostic Tests And Procedures 25
1. Blood testing:..25
2. Stool studies:..26

3. Colonoscopy and sigmoidoscopy: 26

4. Imaging studies: 26

5. Breath testing: 27

6. Food diaries and elimination diets: 27

CHAPTER 3 29

Managing Ibs Through Diet 29

The Role Of Diet In Ibs Management 29

Foods To Avoid 29

1. Foods High in Fermentable Oligosaccharides, Disaccharides, Monosaccharides, and Polyols (FODMAPs): 30

2. Meals that Cause Gas: 30

3. Spicy meals: 30

4. High-Fat Foods: 31

5. Alcohol and Caffeine: 31

Foods That Can Help 32

1. Foods High in Soluble Fiber: 32

2. Low-FODMAP Foods: 32

3. Foods High in Probiotics: 33

4. Lean Protein Sources: 33

5. Herbal Teas: 33

Introduction To Low Fodmap Diet 34

- 1. Phase of Elimination: 35
- 2. Phase of Reintroduction: 35
- 3. Maintenance Phase: 35

CHAPTER 4 37
Lifestyle Modifications For Ibs 37
Stress Management Techniques 37
Exercise And Physical Activity 39
Sleep Hygiene 42

CHAPTER 5 45
Medications For Ibs 45
Over-The-Counter Options 45
- 1. Antidiarrheal Drugs: 45
- 2. Laxatives: 45
- 3. Antispasmodic Drugs: 46
- 4. Antacids: 46
- 5. Fiber Supplements: 46

Prescription Medications 47
- 1. Antidepressants: 47
- 2. Antibiotics: 47
- 3. Serotonin modulators: 48
- 4. Bile Acid Binders: 48

5. Painkillers: 49
Supplements And Probiotics 49
   1. Probiotics: 49
   2. Peppermint Oil: 50
   3. Fiber Supplements: 50
   4. Digestive Enzymes: 50
   5. Fish Oil: 51

CHAPTER 6 53
   Alternative Therapies 53
   Herbal Remedies 53
   The Use Of Acupuncture 55
   The Use Of Hypnosis 57

CHAPTER 7 61
   Coping With Emotional Aspects Of Ibs 61
   Anxiety And Depression Management 61
   Support Groups And Counseling 63

CHAPTER 8 67
   Practical Tips For Everyday Living 67
   Managing Symptoms At Work 67
   Traveling With Ibs 69
   Socializing And Dining Out 71

CHAPTER 9 73
   Ibs And Other Health Conditions............................73
   Ibs And Mental Health 73
   Ibs And Inflammatory Bowel Disease (Ibd) 75
   Ibs And Other Digestive Disorders...........................77

CHAPTER 10 81
   IBS and Gut Health..81
   Understanding Gut Microbiota 81
   How Gut Health Affects Ibs 83
   Probiotics And Prebiotics For Ibs 85

CHAPTER 11 87
   Future Directions And Hope 87
   Advances In Ibs Research 87
   Promising Therapies On The Horizon 90
   Living Well With Ibs: Looking Ahead 92
   CONCLUSION...96

THE END 99

ABOUT THE BOOK

This book, "Irritable Bowel Syndrome (IBS)," is an invaluable resource for anybody dealing with this difficult and sometimes misdiagnosed illness. Its extensive material explores every facet of IBS, providing insightful analysis and useful guidance for symptom management and enhanced quality of life.

Readers learn all there is to know about IBS in Chapter 1, including its diagnosis, kinds, and symptoms, as well as its underlying causes and triggers. Throughout the remainder of the book, making decisions based on this core information is made possible.

The vital subject of diagnosis is covered in detail in Chapter 2, which also outlines the procedures that must be followed, such as taking a patient's medical history, doing a physical examination, and ordering diagnostic tests.

The third chapter of the book, which discusses the significance of nutrition in controlling IBS, is one of its strongest points. The low-FODMAPS diet and trigger food identification are only two examples of how readers may significantly improve symptom management with little dietary changes.

In Chapter 4, lifestyle changes are discussed. Stress reduction, consistent exercise, and getting enough sleep are all emphasized as ways to reduce the symptoms of IBS.

Readers are given guidance on the variety of drugs and supplements available for managing IBS in Chapter 5, enabling them to choose their course of therapy with knowledge.

In Chapter 6, the book delves into alternative therapies, highlighting the possible benefits of acupuncture, hypnosis, and herbal medicines as supplements to traditional medical treatments.

The emotional and practical components of having IBS are covered in Chapters 7 and 8, which also include coping mechanisms for social situations, anxiety, and depression as well as helpful hints for managing day-to-day living.

The book explores the intricate connection between IBS and other medical disorders in Chapter 9, offering helpful information for those who are managing comorbidities.

An in-depth An in-depth discussion of the gut microbiota, probiotics, and prebiotics in the treatment of IBS is found in Chapter 10, which explores the intriguing field of gut health.

In conclusion, Chapter 11 encourages readers to take a proactive approach to managing their IBS while emphasizing recent advancements in the field's research and potential upcoming treatments.

To sum up, "Irritable Bowel Syndrome (IBS)" is a vital tool for everyone dealing with this illness, providing a plethora of information, helpful guidance, and optimism for the future. The all-encompassing information and holistic approach of this book make it an invaluable tool for anybody trying to manage or overcome IBS.

CHAPTER 1

Understanding Irritable Bowel Syndrome (Ibs)

What Is Ibs?

Consider your digestive tract as an intricate network of roads with distinct lanes serving distinct purposes. Imagine now that there are sporadic traffic bottlenecks, delays, and even barricades on this roadway. This resembles the symptoms of irritable bowel syndrome (IBS) in several ways. This gastrointestinal ailment impacts the way your intestines operate, leading to pain, discomfort, and altered bowel patterns.

Fundamentally, IBS is a chronic illness marked by recurrent episodes of pain or discomfort in the abdomen, often combined with constipation or diarrhea. The chronic nature of IBS and the lack of obvious symptoms of illness or injury in the digestive system are what distinguish it. Even while

IBS is common, its precise origin is still unknown, which makes it a challenging conundrum for both patients and medical professionals.

Symptoms Of Ibs

IBS symptoms might vary greatly from person to person in terms of intensity and presentation. The most typical symptoms are gas, bloating, and changed bowel habits in addition to stomach pain or discomfort. While some people may incline more toward constipation, others may predominantly suffer diarrhea. Furthermore, the occurrence and severity of symptoms may vary over time, often brought on by dietary modifications, hormone fluctuations, or stress.

Imagine this: one morning you wake up with a bloated and unpleasant sensation. You could get stomach cramps later in the day, which would need you to make quick visits to the restroom. Your routine may be disturbed by these symptoms, which may have an impact on your job, social life, and general well-being. It is essential to comprehend these symptoms if you want to successfully manage your IBS and enhance your quality of life.

Types Of Ibs

There is no one-size-fits-all kind of IBS; instead, it manifests itself in a variety of ways, each with unique symptoms and difficulties. There are three main forms of IBS:

1. IBS with Constipation (IBS-C): Constipation is the main symptom for those with IBS-C, as the name implies. They could have hard, lumpy, or challenging-to-pass stools, and they might have fewer bowel motions than normal.

2. IBS with diarrhea (IBS-D): On the other hand, diarrhea episodes are common in IBS-D. There may

be urgency, loose, watery stools, as well as an inability to regulate bowel motions.

3. Mixed IBS (IBS-M): IBS may cause a variety of symptoms for some unlucky people, with constipation and diarrhea alternating. Because it adds an unpredictable aspect to bowel movements, this rollercoaster ride may be quite difficult to handle.

Determining the particular subtype of IBS you have is essential to customizing your treatment regimen and successfully controlling your symptoms. Remember that people may change over time between different subtypes, which would add still another level of intricacy to the illness.

Causes And Triggers

Examining the complex network of causes and triggers of IBS is necessary to unravel its enigma. The genesis of IBS symptoms is yet unknown, however, several variables are thought to have a role in their emergence and aggravation.

1. **Stomach Dysfunction:** According to a widely accepted idea, irregularities in the interaction between the stomach, brain, and neurological system are the cause of IBS. Increased pain sensitivity, altered motility, and aberrant reactions to stress and food may result from this disorder.

2. **Dietary Factors:** Your food may both cause and perhaps alleviate IBS symptoms. It is crucial to keep this in mind. There is evidence that some meals and drinks, including those high in caffeine, alcohol, artificial sweeteners, and spicy foods, might exacerbate symptoms in certain people. However, many IBS patients have found that using a low-FODMAP diet, which restricts certain kinds of carbs, might help to lessen their symptoms.

3. **Stress and Mental Health:** It's no secret that stress may negatively impact every part of your body, including your digestive system. Stress and worry may either cause or exacerbate symptoms for those who have IBS, leading to a vicious cycle of physical pain and emotional suffering. Acquiring knowledge of stress-reduction methods like deep breathing exercises, mindfulness, and meditation may be very helpful in controlling the symptoms of IBS.

4. **Gut Microbiota:** Your digestive system's health is greatly influenced by the billions of microorganisms that live in your gut. Various gastrointestinal illnesses, including IBS, have been linked to imbalances in these microbial ecosystems. Beneficial bacteria called probiotics have gained attention as a possible therapeutic intervention for microbial balance restoration and symptom relief in some IBS patients.

Healthcare professionals may create individualized treatment programs targeted at treating the underlying causes and triggers of IBS by figuring out the complex interactions between these variables. A holistic strategy that includes dietary adjustments, stress management strategies, and targeted treatments may help people better manage their symptoms and enhance their overall quality of life, even if there isn't a one-size-fits-all answer.

CHAPTER 2

Diagnosing Ibs

Criteria For Diagnosis

Irritable Bowel Syndrome (IBS) diagnosis requires a thorough assessment based on predetermined standards. For this, the Rome criteria are often used. These criteria state that to be diagnosed with IBS, a person must have recurring stomach pain or discomfort for at least three days per month over the previous three months, with the beginning of symptoms occurring at least six months before the diagnosis, and be linked to two or more of the following:

1. Enhanced by defecating.

2. beginning correlated with a shift in the frequency of stools.

3. Beginning coincided with a change in the stool's shape or appearance.

These standards provide a consistent framework for diagnosis and assist in distinguishing IBS from other gastrointestinal illnesses. It's important to remember that these standards are not rigid and should be interpreted in light of further clinical data.

Medical History And Physical Examination

Examining the patient physically and obtaining a complete medical history are the initial steps in diagnosing IBS. Healthcare professionals will ask about the patient's symptoms, including frequency, duration, and severity of abdominal pain or discomfort, along with any related symptoms like dietary changes, stress levels, altered bowel habits, or a family history of gastrointestinal disorders, during the medical history.

During a physical examination, the abdomen may be palpated to feel for lumps, distension, or discomfort. To check for anomalies in the rectum or anus, the medical professional may also do a digital rectal examination. We will also assess any other systemic symptoms or indicators that could point to underlying issues.

Diagnostic Tests And Procedures

Although there isn't a single test that can be used to identify IBS, diagnostic procedures and tests may be carried out to rule out other diseases and validate the diagnosis. These examinations might consist of:

1. **Blood testing:** Blood tests may be carried out to look for indications of inflammation, infection, or other abnormalities that could point to the presence of an underlying illness, such as thyroid problems, inflammatory bowel disease (IBD), or celiac disease.

2. **Stool studies:** Blood, pathogens (such as bacteria, viruses, or parasites), and anomalies in the digestive system may all be found in stool samples. These analyses can be used to diagnose diseases including infection, inflammation, or malabsorption.

3. **Colonoscopy and sigmoidoscopy:** These procedures include the visual inspection of the lining of the colon and rectum for abnormalities, such as inflammation, ulcers, or polyps, by inserting a flexible tube with a camera into the colon (colonoscopy) or lower section of the colon (sigmoidoscopy). These tests are very helpful in excluding diseases like colorectal cancer and inflammatory bowel disease.

4. **Imaging studies:** To view the digestive system and find structural abnormalities or other disorders that could be causing symptoms, imaging

tests like abdominal ultrasound, CT scan, or MRI may be carried out.

5. Breath testing: Breath tests may be used to identify digestive anomalies such as lactose intolerance or bacterial overgrowth, which can exacerbate the symptoms of IBS.

6. Food diaries and elimination diets: Under the supervision of a healthcare professional, keeping a food diary or following an elimination diet may help pinpoint certain foods or dietary triggers that worsen IBS symptoms.

These diagnostic techniques and tests assist medical professionals in confirming the diagnosis of IBS, ruling out other disorders that present with similar symptoms, and creating a treatment plan that is suitable and customized for each patient.

CHAPTER 3

Managing Ibs Through Diet

The Role Of Diet In Ibs Management

The management of Irritable Bowel Syndrome (IBS) is heavily influenced by diet. The intensity of your symptoms may be greatly influenced by what you eat, even if it might not be the only cause of IBS. You can take charge of your IBS and live a more pleasant life if you know which meals make you uncomfortable and which ones calm your digestive system.

Foods To Avoid

It is advisable to limit or stay away from certain meals since they are known to exacerbate the symptoms of IBS.

Among them are:

1. **Foods High in Fermentable Oligosaccharides, Disaccharides, Monosaccharides, and Polyols (FODMAPs):** Some individuals may have trouble digesting these kinds of carbs. Onions, garlic, wheat, mangoes, onions, and various dairy products are foods rich in fructooligosaccharides (FODMAPS). For those with IBS, these foods may cause bloating, gas, and discomfort in the abdomen.

2. **Meals that Cause Gas:** Certain meals have a reputation for causing the digestive system to overproduce gas, which may cause bloating and discomfort. These consist of cabbage, beans, lentils, and fizzy drinks. Reducing the amount of these items you eat may assist with symptoms.

3. **Spicy meals:** For those with IBS, spicy meals may irritate the digestive system and cause symptoms including diarrhea and stomach discomfort.

Relief may come from avoiding or consuming less spicy foods, such as chili peppers and hot sauce.

4. **High-Fat Foods:** Saturated and trans fats in particular might exacerbate the symptoms of IBS. These meals may cause constipation and bloating by slowing down digestion. Reducing the amount of fried meals, fatty meats, and creamy sauces you consume may help control your symptoms.

5. **Alcohol and Caffeine:** Both substances can agitate the digestive system and promote bowel motions, which may exacerbate diarrhea and pain in the abdomen in people with IBS. It could be good to cut down on your alcohol, tea, and coffee consumption.

The frequency and intensity of your IBS symptoms may be greatly decreased by recognizing and avoiding certain trigger foods.

Foods That Can Help

While certain foods might make symptoms of IBS worse, others can help and promote digestive health. Including these items in your diet might help reduce pain and enhance general health:

1. **Foods High in Soluble Fiber:** Soluble fiber may relieve the constipation and diarrhea brought on by IBS and aid in the regulation of bowel movements. Oats, barley, psyllium husk, and fruits like bananas and berries are good sources of soluble fiber. You may aid in bettering digestive function by progressively increasing your soluble fiber intake.

2. **Low-FODMAP Foods:** It has been shown that many people have a reduction in IBS symptoms when they adhere to a low-FODMAP diet, which consists of reducing foods rich in fermentable carbs. Rice, potatoes, carrots, spinach, and dairy products without lactose are examples of foods low in

FODMAPs. It is advised to collaborate with a dietician or healthcare provider to safely and successfully follow a Low FODMAP diet.

3. **Foods High in Probiotics:** Probiotics are good bacteria that support gut health and may help reduce the symptoms of irritable bowel syndrome. Probiotic-rich foods include kimchi, sauerkraut, kefir, and yogurt. By including these items in your diet, you may enhance digestive health and help your gut bacteria return to equilibrium.

4. **Lean Protein Sources:** You may get the vital nutrients you need without aggravating your IBS symptoms by choosing lean protein sources like fish, chicken, tofu, and lentils. In general, these protein sources are less prone to upset your stomach and are simpler to digest.

5. **Herbal Teas:** Some herbal teas, including chamomile and peppermint, have calming qualities

that might help reduce bloating and other symptoms of IBS. After a meal, sipping a warm cup of herbal tea may help relieve tension and encourage calmness.

You may promote digestive health and lessen the burden of IBS on your everyday life by including these gut-friendly items in your diet.

Introduction To Low Fodmap Diet

A specific dietary strategy called the Low FODMAP diet aims to control IBS symptoms by limiting the intake of particular carbohydrates called FODMAPs. Because FODMAPs are osmotic and fermentable, they may pull water into the intestines where gut bacteria might ferment them, causing symptoms in sensitive people including gas, bloating, and changed bowel patterns.

There are three primary stages to the Low FODMAP diet:

1. Phase of Elimination: Foods rich in FODMAPs are cut out of the diet for a duration of two to six weeks during this phase. This relieves IBS symptoms and aids in identifying trigger foods.

2. Phase of Reintroduction: Following the elimination stage, modest amounts of each FODMAP are reintroduced one at a time to gauge tolerance. This stage makes it possible to customize the diet and helps determine which FODMAPs cause discomfort.

3. Maintenance Phase: After identifying the trigger foods, the diet is modified to cut out just those that are rich in FODMAPs and produce symptoms. Maintaining symptom management while taking advantage of a diverse and well-balanced diet is the aim of this phase.

Careful preparation and direction from a medical practitioner or registered dietitian with expertise in treating IBS is necessary while adhering to the Low FODMAP diet. When on this limited diet, it is important to reduce the danger of nutritional shortages and guarantee proper nutrient intake.

Individuals with IBS can take proactive measures to enhance their digestive health and quality of life by learning how diet plays a role in managing their condition and putting strategies like gut-friendly food incorporation, avoiding trigger foods, and researching dietary interventions like the Low FODMAP diet into practice.

CHAPTER 4

Lifestyle Modifications For Ibs

Stress Management Techniques

For those who suffer from Irritable Bowel Syndrome (IBS), stress management is crucial since stress may aggravate symptoms including bloating, stomach discomfort, and altered bowel patterns. Your quality of life may be greatly enhanced by incorporating stress management practices into your everyday routine.

Deep breathing exercises are one useful stress-reduction method. By triggering the body's relaxation response, deep breathing helps lessen the physiological impacts of stress. To engage in deep breathing, take a few slow breaths via your nose, hold them, and then slowly release them through your mouth.

Repeat this exercise many times while paying attention to your breathing and letting your body relax.

Progressive muscle relaxation is another useful method (PMR). To induce relaxation and lessen muscular tension, PMR entails tensing and then releasing various muscle groups in your body. For a few seconds, tense the muscles in your feet. Then, progressively go up your body, tensing and releasing each muscle group.

Stress reduction is another advantage of mindfulness meditation. Reducing stress and anxiety may be achieved by practicing mindfulness, which is focusing attention on the here and now without passing judgment. Locate a peaceful area to sit comfortably, shut your eyes, and concentrate on your breathing or a particular bodily experience. Gently return your focus to the here and now when your thoughts stray, without passing judgment.

It's crucial to include stress-relieving activities in your everyday routine in addition to these strategies. Take part in things you like doing, including reading, listening to music, going on nature walks, or taking up a hobby. Make self-care activities that encourage relaxation and well-being a priority, and plan frequent breaks throughout the day to rest and rejuvenate.

You may significantly lessen the negative effects of stress on your IBS symptoms and enhance your general quality of life by implementing stress management strategies into your daily routine.

Exercise And Physical Activity

In addition to helping to manage the symptoms of Irritable Bowel Syndrome (IBS), regular exercise and physical activity can improve general health and wellbeing. Exercise eases stress, balances mood, lessens gas and bloating and improves bowel function.

Walking, running, cycling, or swimming are examples of aerobic activity that might help encourage bowel movements and ease constipation, a typical symptom of IBS. To reap the advantages, try to get in at least 30 minutes of moderate-intensity aerobic activity most days of the week.

Strength training activities might be good to include in your program in addition to cardiovascular activity. It is possible to enhance bowel movement and lessen symptoms like bloating and pain in the belly by strengthening the muscles of the abdomen and pelvic floor.

Another great alternative for those with IBS is yoga. Yoga promotes relaxation, lowers stress levels, and improves digestion via the use of physical postures, breathing techniques, and meditation. By encouraging the digestive system and easing abdominal strain, certain yoga positions, such as twists and moderate stretches, may help reduce the symptoms of IBS.

It's crucial to pay attention to your body and begin a fitness program gradually, particularly if you've never worked out before or have been inactive for some time. As your fitness level rises, gradually increase the length and intensity of your exercises. To maintain your activity level, nourish your body with healthy meals and drink enough of water.

Regular physical activity and exercise may help control the symptoms of IBS, promote general health, and improve quality of life.

Sleep Hygiene

Getting enough sleep is crucial for maintaining general health and well-being, which includes controlling Irritable Bowel Syndrome (IBS) symptoms. IBS symptoms including bloating, irregular bowel movements, and stomach discomfort may be made worse by poor sleep patterns. For those who have IBS, maintaining proper sleep hygiene is thus essential.

Promoting good sleep patterns requires establishing a regular sleep routine. To keep your body's internal clock in check, try to go to bed and get up at the same time every day—even on the weekends. Establish a calming evening routine that involves taking a warm bath, reading a book, or other relaxation methods to let your body know it's time to wind down.

Improving the quality of sleep may also include setting up a cozy sleeping space. Make sure your bedroom is cold, quiet, and dark. You should also get pillows and a comfy mattress to promote healthy sleep. Reduce the amount of time spent in front of computers, tablets, and cellphones before bed since the blue light they generate might interfere with sleep cycles.

Steer clear of coffee, nicotine, and alcohol just before bed since these may disrupt sleep and make IBS symptoms worse. Instead, to help you relax and go to sleep, use warm milk or herbal teas.

Consult your healthcare physician if your IBS symptoms are keeping you from sleeping. They may provide direction and suggest methods to enhance the quality of your sleep, such as dietary changes, medication adjustments, or a recommendation to see a sleep expert.

Making sleep a priority and emphasizing proper sleep hygiene can help you better manage the symptoms of irritable bowel syndrome and enhance your general health.

CHAPTER 5

Medications For Ibs

Over-The-Counter Options

Some of the symptoms of Irritable Bowel Syndrome (IBS) may be relieved with over-the-counter (OTC) solutions. The facts that these drugs are readily available and do not needs a prescription make them an ideal option for a lot of people with IBS.

1. **Antidiarrheal Drugs:** These drugs may help control bowel movements if diarrhea is a common symptom of your IBS. These drugs relieve the urgency and frequency of frequent bowel movements by slowing down the intestines' motility.

2. **Laxatives:** On the other hand, they may be used to encourage bowel motions if constipation is the primary problem. Laxatives come in a variety of forms, such as bulk-forming, stimulant, and osmotic

laxatives. It's important to choose the appropriate kind depending on your symptoms and, if necessary, seek medical advice.

3. **Antispasmodic Drugs:** These drugs relieve intestinal muscular tension, which helps lessen the cramping and discomfort in the abdomen that are linked to IBS. They are especially beneficial for those whose symptoms include cramps or spasms.

4. **Antacids:** By neutralizing stomach acid, antacids may help those with IBS who also suffer from acid reflux or heartburn. This may assist in easing upper gastrointestinal pain.

5. **Fiber Supplements:** For IBS patients with a predominance of diarrhea or constipation, fiber supplements may be helpful. By making the stool more substantial and encouraging regularity, they may aid in controlling bowel motions. To avoid exacerbating symptoms, it is necessary to

begin with moderate dosages and increase consumption gradually.

Prescription Medications

If managing IBS symptoms with over-the-counter choices proves to be inadequate, a healthcare professional may prescribe prescription drugs. These drugs are designed to address certain IBS symptoms or underlying reasons, and they are often more effective.

1. **Antidepressants:** Several antidepressant drugs, especially selective serotonin reuptake inhibitors (SSRIs) and tricyclic antidepressants (TCAs), be useful in treating the symptoms of IBS. They work by changing the brain's and the gut's levels of neurotransmitters, which may lessen pain and enhance bowel movement.

2. **Antibiotics:** Small intestinal bacterial overgrowth (SIBO), a condition that may worsen the symptoms

of irritable bowel syndrome (IBS), may sometimes be treated with antibiotics. Antibiotics assist in getting rid of too many germs in the small intestine, which helps some people feel better.

3. Serotonin modulators: Drugs like alosetron and tegaserod, which target serotonin receptors in the stomach, may help control bowel movements and lessen symptoms like discomfort and diarrhea. Due to possible adverse effects, these drugs are usually only prescribed to those with severe IBS symptoms who have not improved with previous therapies.

4. Bile Acid Binders: People with bile acid malabsorption, which may aggravate diarrhea in IBS patients, may be administered bile acid binders, such as cholestyramine and colesevelam. To stop extra bile acids from irritating the colon and producing symptoms, these drugs attach to them in the gut.

5. **Painkillers:** Short-term prescription painkillers may be recommended for those who are suffering from excruciating stomach pain. Although these drugs may provide short-term comfort, long-term use is usually not advised because of the possibility of dependency and other negative consequences.

Supplements And Probiotics

Probiotics and supplements can help control IBS symptoms in addition to prescription drugs. These products include a variety of ingredients that may help reduce symptoms and enhance gut health.

1. **Probiotics:** Good for digestive health, probiotics are live bacteria and yeasts. They can aid in reestablishing the proper balance of gut flora and alleviate symptoms like gas, bloating, and irregular bowel movements. Probiotic supplements come in a variety of forms, such as powders, capsules, and fermented foods like kefir and yogurt.

2. **Peppermint Oil:** Research has demonstrated that using peppermint oil as a natural remedy can help reduce symptoms of IBS, specifically bloating and pain in the abdomen. It functions by lowering inflammation and calming the intestinal muscles. For relief, peppermint oil capsules can be taken orally and are available as a dietary supplement.

3. **Fiber Supplements:** As previously indicated, by encouraging regular bowel movements and averting constipation or diarrhea, fiber supplements can help manage the symptoms of IBS. Supplements containing soluble fiber, like methylcellulose or psyllium husk, are frequently advised because they are less likely than insoluble fiber to result in gas and bloating.

4. **Digestive Enzymes:** Some IBS sufferers experience problems breaking down specific foods, which can result in symptoms like gas and

bloating. Digestive discomfort can be minimized by taking supplements that contain digestive enzymes, which aid in the more efficient breakdown of proteins, fats, and carbs.

5. Fish Oil: The anti-inflammatory qualities of omega-3 fatty acids, which are present in fish oil supplements, may help people with IBS, especially those who have inflammatory bowel disease (IBD). While more research is required to determine whether fish oil is particularly effective for IBS, some people report relief from symptoms like diarrhea and abdominal pain.

Irritable Bowel Syndrome (IBS) management frequently necessitates a multimodal strategy that may include dietary adjustments, medication, or supplement therapy, as well as lifestyle changes. Working closely with a healthcare provider is essential to creating a customized treatment plan that takes into account your unique needs and symptoms. People with IBS can find relief and enhance their quality of life by investigating the different medication options, such as over-the-counter remedies, prescription medications, supplements, and probiotics.

CHAPTER 6

Alternative Therapies

Herbal Remedies

For centuries, people have used herbal remedies to treat a variety of health issues, such as digestive disorders like Irritable Bowel Syndrome (IBS). These all-natural, plant-based products are a kinder option for treating IBS symptoms than prescription drugs. Herbal remedies can address multiple symptoms at once, providing a comprehensive approach to treatment, which is one of their main advantages.

A popular herbal treatment for IBS, peppermint oil is well-known for relieving pain and discomfort in the abdomen. It reduces bloating, eases spasms, and relaxes the muscles of the gastrointestinal tract. Enteric-coated tablets or capsules containing peppermint oil are frequently used to guarantee the oil reaches the intestines undamaged and can start working.

Ginger is another herb that is frequently used for IBS. Ginger relieves symptoms like nausea and indigestion by soothing the digestive tract and having anti-inflammatory qualities. It can be drunk raw, brewed as a tea, or taken as a supplement.

Because of its well-known calming qualities, chamomile is frequently used to reduce stress and anxiety, which can worsen the symptoms of IBS. As an herbal remedy, chamomile tea helps ease digestive tract muscle tension, which lessens spasms and encourages regular bowel movements.

Apart from these herbs, fennel, turmeric, and aloe vera have also demonstrated potential in the management of irritable bowel syndrome symptoms. Herbal remedies may interact with other medications or exacerbate certain symptoms, so it's important to speak with a healthcare provider before adding them to your IBS treatment plan.

The Use Of Acupuncture

Thin needles are inserted into predetermined body points during acupuncture, an age-old Chinese medical practice, to reduce pain and encourage healing. Acupuncture has become known as a complementary therapy for several ailments, including IBS, despite its unusual appearance.

Acupuncture is based on the theory that it helps the body's qi, or energy flow, to be more balanced. Acupuncture for IBS seeks to balance the digestive system's operation, thereby mitigating symptoms like bloating, diarrhea, and constipation.

Acupuncture may be beneficial for people with IBS, according to several studies. For instance, a review of clinical trials revealed that acupuncture improved

IBS symptoms more than sham acupuncture, which involves inserting needles at non-acupuncture sites.

In a typical 30- to 60-minute session, the acupuncturist will insert needles into predetermined body points, frequently concentrating on the lower back and abdomen. Acupuncture is often described as a soothing and painless procedure; some patients even report feeling immediate relief from IBS symptoms.

Even though acupuncture is generally regarded as safe when administered by a licensed professional, not everyone may benefit from it. Before receiving acupuncture treatment, people with specific medical conditions or those taking blood thinners should speak with their healthcare provider.

The Use Of Hypnosis

Through the use of hypnosis to create a state of intense relaxation and focused attention, hypnotherapy is a therapeutic approach that enables people to access their subconscious minds. Hypnotherapy for IBS seeks to address the underlying psychological factors that may contribute to the condition to alleviate symptoms.

Elevated stress, anxiety, or depression are common in IBS sufferers, and this can make symptoms worse. The method by which hypnotherapy reduces the frequency and intensity of IBS flare-ups is by assisting patients in recognizing and addressing these psychological triggers.

In a hypnotherapy session, a qualified therapist will lead the patient into a deeply relaxed state and offer helpful visualizations and affirmations regarding their IBS symptoms. These recommendations aim to rewire the subconscious, fostering composure and control over the digestive tract.

Studies have indicated that hypnotherapy can be very successful in reducing the symptoms of irritable bowel syndrome (IBS), with notable improvements noted in bloating, abdominal pain, and bowel habits after treatment. Many people also mention long-lasting advantages, with hypnotherapy's effects continuing long after treatment is over.

It's crucial to remember that hypnotherapy should only be administered by a licensed, skilled therapist with experience treating IBS. Furthermore, even though hypnotherapy is generally safe, not everyone is a good candidate for it, especially if they have certain mental health issues or are hesitant to participate completely in the process.

In conclusion, those looking for all-natural ways to manage their IBS symptoms may find that complementary therapies like acupuncture, hypnosis, and herbal medicines are promising. But before implementing these therapies into your treatment plan, it's crucial to proceed cautiously and speak with a medical expert. When combined with a tailored approach and appropriate guidance, alternative therapies can significantly enhance the quality of life for individuals suffering from irritable bowel syndrome.

CHAPTER 7

Coping With Emotional Aspects Of Ibs

Anxiety And Depression Management

Irritable bowel syndrome (IBS) sufferers frequently experience anxiety and depression. These feelings may be influenced by the erratic nature of symptoms, their influence on day-to-day activities, and the uncertainty surrounding the onset of new symptoms. Nonetheless, there are methods for controlling the melancholy and anxiety brought on by IBS.

A good strategy is to practice mindfulness meditation. This technique, which entails focusing on the here and now without passing judgment, can ease tension and encourage calm. People with IBS can learn to relax and reduce anxiety by concentrating on their breathing or body sensations.

Cognitive-behavioral therapy is another useful method (CBT). The goal of CBT is to recognize and alter harmful thought patterns and behavior patterns that fuel anxiety and depression. With the help of professional therapy sessions, people can acquire coping mechanisms and cultivate a more optimistic perspective on handling their IBS symptoms.

Exercise regularly can be very helpful in managing anxiety and depression in addition to these therapies. Engaging in physical activity can help lower stress levels and release endorphins, which are naturally occurring mood enhancers. On mental health, even small actions like doing yoga or going for regular walks can be beneficial.

In addition, controlling anxiety and depression requires eating a balanced diet and getting adequate sleep. Caffeine and alcohol are two foods and beverages that can worsen IBS symptoms and cause mood swings. A balanced diet and good sleep hygiene are two ways that people with IBS can improve their general mental health.

Finally, people with IBS must ask friends, family, or a mental health professional for support. Speaking about their emotions and experiences can help people feel less alone and isolated by validating and encouraging them. Support groups can also provide helpful guidance and coping mechanisms for managing the psychological aspects of IBS.

People with IBS can enhance their overall quality of life and more effectively manage their anxiety and depression by adopting these techniques into their daily routines.

Support Groups And Counseling

For people with irritable bowel syndrome, support groups, and counseling can be quite helpful (IBS). These platforms provide a secure and compassionate space where people can talk about their experiences, get support, and pick up coping mechanisms from others going through comparable struggles.

Getting involved in a support group can give people with IBS a feeling of belonging and community. Feelings of loneliness and isolation can be lessened by interacting with people who are aware of the challenges that come with having IBS every day. Furthermore, getting inspiration and hope comes from learning about the accomplishments and experiences of other group members.

Support groups provide flexibility for people to participate based on their schedules and preferences. They can meet in person or virtually. Members of IBS-focused social media groups and online forums can interact with people worldwide, offering a variety of viewpoints and support.

To help manage the emotional aspects of IBS, individual counseling can be helpful in addition to support groups. A qualified therapist can assist people in exploring their emotions, creating coping mechanisms, and addressing any underlying problems that may be causing them to experience anxiety or depression.

Techniques like mindfulness meditation, cognitive-behavioral therapy (CBT), or customized relaxation exercises may be used in counseling sessions. Attending frequent sessions can help people better understand their feelings and actions, develop useful coping mechanisms, and adopt a more optimistic approach to controlling their IBS symptoms.

Finding a support group or counselor who fits their needs and preferences and with whom they feel comfortable is crucial for people with IBS. Having a network of peers and professionals who are supportive can be very helpful in managing the emotional challenges of living with IBS, whether one seeks support in person or online.

In conclusion, for people with IBS who are looking for a sense of community, coping mechanisms, and emotional support, support groups and counseling are invaluable resources. Through collaborating with skilled professionals and forming connections with like-minded individuals, people can enhance their general well-being and effectively manage symptoms of depression and anxiety.

CHAPTER 8

Practical Tips For Everyday Living

Managing Symptoms At Work

It can be difficult to navigate the workplace while managing the symptoms of irritable bowel syndrome (IBS), but comfort and productivity can be maintained with a few useful techniques. To start, communication is essential. Think about discussing your condition with your employer or the HR department, outlining how it might impact your work, and requiring any necessary accommodations. This can entail having access to a private restroom or having flexible working hours.

Additionally, since stress can make IBS symptoms worse, it's critical to control your stress levels. Stress-reduction methods like deep breathing exercises, meditation, or taking quick breaks during the day can be incorporated to help reduce symptoms and enhance general well-being. Furthermore, figuring out how to arrange your workload and prioritize your tasks can help you feel less stressed and overwhelmed.

Making your meals and snacks can help you stick to a diet because you can manage the ingredients and serving sizes. Choose foods that are simple to digest, like whole grains, fruits, vegetables, and lean proteins. Caffeine, spicy foods, and high-fat meals are examples of triggers. You may also want to keep a food journal to monitor the impact of various foods on your symptoms.

Finally, remember that it's okay to take breaks when necessary. Give yourself a moment to step away from your desk and engage in some relaxation exercises if you're feeling uncomfortable or if your symptoms are flare-ups. Never forget that taking care of yourself should always come first.

During the workday, don't be afraid to give self-care priority.

Traveling With Ibs

IBS requires additional planning and preparation when traveling, but with the right strategy, it's completely manageable. First, do some advanced research on your destination to find lodging options and restrooms that are close by and can accommodate your needs. This can ensure that you feel comfortable the entire trip and help reduce anxiety.

Make sure to pack essentials for your trip, such as prescription drugs, dietary supplements, and any particular foods or snacks you know won't upset your stomach. For peace of mind, it's also a good idea to bring along a travel-sized toilet kit that includes supplies like hand sanitizer, wet wipes, and toilet paper.

Drink plenty of water and try your best to keep to your regular eating schedule while traveling. Light, easily digestible snacks are preferable to heavy meals or trigger foods before and during travel. If you're flying, be aware of how cabin altitude and air pressure changes may impact your symptoms. You may also want to ask for an aisle seat to facilitate easier access to the restrooms.

Pace yourself and pay attention to your body's cues while exploring your destination. Never be afraid to take breaks and rest when necessary if you're feeling worn out or if your symptoms are getting worse. To ensure that you can enjoy your travels without experiencing additional stress, it's also helpful to plan activities and outings that allow for flexibility and convenient access to restroom facilities.

Socializing And Dining Out

It's not impossible to have an active social life and go out to eat when you have IBS. You can still enjoy meals and social gatherings with friends and family if you plan and communicate. First and foremost, don't be afraid to let your friends know about any dietary limitations and any unique requirements about your health. It can help ease your anxiety or discomfort, and most people will be accommodating and understanding.

When going out to eat, check ahead for restaurants that will accommodate your dietary requirements. These days, a lot of places have low-FODMAPS, dairy-free, and gluten-free menu options, which makes it simpler to find foods that won't aggravate your symptoms. You should not be afraid to ask your server for clarification if you have questions about any ingredients or preparation techniques.

Eating smaller, more frequent meals throughout the day is also a good idea as opposed to indulging in large, heavy meals that may make symptoms worse. Pay attention to the amount you eat and pay attention to your body's signals of hunger and fullness. Additionally, if you're not sure what options are available at a specific restaurant, think about packing snacks or even a small meal substitute.

Consider spending more time with your friends and family during social events than just the food. Take part in activities or conversations that divert your attention from any discomfort you may be experiencing, and don't be afraid to ask to be excused if you need to go somewhere to relax or take a break. Recall that, even in social situations, it's acceptable to put your health and well-being first.

CHAPTER 9

Ibs And Other Health Conditions

Ibs And Mental Health

Gastrointestinal problems and mental health problems often coexist; IBS is only one example. The gut-brain axis, a network of two-way communication between the brain and the gastrointestinal system, plays a significant role in this. IBS is uncomfortable and unpredictable, and stress, worry, and depression may exacerbate symptoms. It can also cause mental health problems.

When treating IBS, it's important to consider how it impacts mental health and vice versa. IBS symptoms as well as related mental health problems may be managed with the use of strategies including stress management, mindfulness, and cognitive-behavioral therapy

(CBT). By focusing on the interaction between ideas, feelings, and actions, these methods enable people to create coping mechanisms.

Moreover, dietary and lifestyle changes that promote a balanced diet, frequent exercise, and enough sleep might improve mental and gastrointestinal health. Creating a solid support system with friends, family, or support groups may also be a great way to get emotional assistance.

It can be required to seek professional assistance from a therapist or psychiatrist in situations when mental health issues have a substantial influence on day-to-day functioning. Medication to control anxiety or depression or therapies like cognitive behavioral therapy (CBT) customized for IBS may provide relief and enhance overall quality of life.

Comprehensive treatment of IBS requires an understanding of the relationship between IBS and mental health. People may better manage the difficulties presented by this complicated ailment and enhance their general well-being by treating both components holistically.

Ibs And Inflammatory Bowel Disease (Ibd)

Although the symptoms of inflammatory bowel disease (IBD) and IBS are somewhat similar, they are two separate illnesses with different underlying causes and therapeutic modalities. IBD includes diseases like Crohn's disease and ulcerative colitis that cause the gastrointestinal tract to become inflamed over time, whereas IBS is defined by symptoms related to the functioning of the intestine that are not associated with inflammation or structural abnormalities.

But it's also common for people with IBD to have IBS-like symptoms, or "IBS-like symptoms in IBD." These symptoms, which can include bloating, altered bowel habits, and abdominal pain, can occur as a result of overlapping pathophysiological mechanisms or the effects of IBD treatments.

Making the distinction between IBS and IBD is essential for the right kind of care. While IBD necessitates medical intervention to reduce inflammation and avoid problems, IBS care focuses on symptom alleviation and quality of life enhancement by dietary adjustments, lifestyle changes, and medication targeted at specific symptoms.

Dual diagnoses of IBD and IBS might occur sometimes, requiring a multidisciplinary treatment comprising nutritionists, gastroenterologists, and mental health specialists. Treatment regimens may be designed to target both problems simultaneously to maximize results and provide complete care.

For people with both IBS and IBD, regular monitoring and discussion with healthcare professionals are crucial since symptoms and treatment requirements might change over time. A proactive approach to treatment and a knowledge of the interrelationships between these disorders may help people better manage their general health and gastrointestinal health.

Ibs And Other Digestive Disorders

Co-occurring digestive diseases with IBS might make diagnosis and treatment more challenging. IBS symptoms may coexist with other illnesses such as small intestinal bacterial overgrowth (SIBO), celiac disease, and gastroesophageal reflux disease (GERD), which can complicate diagnosis and therapy.

Heartburn and regurgitation are two symptoms of GERD, which is defined by acid reflux from the stomach into the esophagus. These symptoms may coexist with those of IBS, including bloating and abdominal discomfort. Similar to IBS presentations, gastrointestinal symptoms including diarrhea and bloating may be present in celiac disease, an autoimmune disorder brought on by gluten consumption.

Abdominal discomfort, bloating, and changes in bowel habits are some of the symptoms of IBS that may potentially be mistaken for small intestinal bacterial overgrowth (SIBO), a condition in which there is an overabundance of bacteria in the small intestine. Specialized testing, such as breath tests or small bowel aspirates, is sometimes necessary to differentiate between SIBO and IBS to verify the existence of bacterial overgrowth.

A thorough strategy customized to each patient's requirements is necessary for managing IBS in addition to other digestive diseases. This might include taking specific drugs to relieve certain symptoms in addition to dietary changes, such as avoiding trigger foods or following a gluten-free diet in the case of celiac disease.

For a proper diagnosis and efficient treatment, gastroenterologists must work in tandem with other experts, such as nutritionists and allergy specialists. Healthcare professionals may maximize results and enhance patients' quality of life by treating IBS and coexisting digestive diseases in a coordinated way.

Individuals who are aware of the possible overlap between IBS and other digestive problems are better able to advocate for comprehensive treatment and thorough assessment.

CHAPTER 10

IBS and Gut Health

Understanding Gut Microbiota

The complex ecology of bacteria that live in your digestive tract is known as the gut microbiota, also known as the gut flora or gut microbiome. These microorganisms, which include bacteria, viruses, fungi, and other microbes, are essential for many body processes, such as metabolism, digestion, and immunity.

There is a varied and well-balanced colony of bacteria in a healthy gut. However, in patients with IBS, there may be an imbalance or dysbiosis in the gut microbiota, where some kinds of bacteria dominate while others are less numerous. The symptoms of IBS, including diarrhea, constipation, bloating, and stomach discomfort, may be exacerbated by this imbalance.

The makeup of the gut microbiota may be influenced by several things, such as stress, drugs, nutrition, and lifestyle choices. For instance, dysbiosis may result from a diet heavy in processed foods and low in fiber, which upsets the equilibrium of gut flora. In a similar vein, long-term stress may potentially change the makeup of the gut microbiota and worsen IBS symptoms.

To create successful treatment plans, it is important to comprehend the function of gut bacteria in IBS. It could be able to help IBS sufferers with their symptoms and enhance their general gut health by bringing the gut microbiome back into equilibrium.

How Gut Health Affects Ibs

The development and treatment of IBS are significantly influenced by the state of your digestive system. In addition to acting as a barrier to keep toxic compounds out of circulation, a healthy gut lining is necessary for optimal digestion and nutrient absorption.

The gut lining of people with IBS may be affected, which may result in increased permeability, or "leaky gut." When the gut lining is compromised, toxins, bacteria, and undigested food particles can seep into the circulation, inciting inflammation and an immunological response. This inflammation may exacerbate the symptoms of IBS and add to the chronic nature of the illness.

Furthermore, a typical feature of IBS patients is disruptions in gut motility or the passage of food through the digestive system. Symptoms of this dysregulation include constipation, diarrhea, and irregular bowel movements.

Moreover, a key factor in IBS is the gut-brain axis, a system of two-way communication between the stomach and the brain. IBS symptoms might worsen when stress and emotions affect intestinal sensitivity and motility. On the other hand, gastrointestinal problems may sometimes set off worry and stress, leading to a vicious cycle.

Developing thorough treatment plans requires an understanding of the complex link between intestinal health and IBS. For those with IBS, improving gut health via targeted medications, dietary changes, and stress reduction strategies may help reduce symptoms and enhance overall quality of life.

Probiotics And Prebiotics For Ibs

Two categories of dietary supplements that may support healthy gut flora and lessen IBS symptoms are probiotics and prebiotics.

Probiotics are living bacteria that provide the host health benefits when taken in sufficient quantities. By lowering inflammation, enhancing gut barrier function, and preventing the development of pathogenic bacteria, these beneficial bacteria may aid in the restoration of the gut microbiota's equilibrium. Numerous probiotic strains, such as Lactobacillus, Bifidobacterium, and Saccharomyces, have been investigated for their possible function in treating IBS symptoms.

Contrarily, prebiotics are indigestible fibers that feed the good bacteria in the stomach. Prebiotics may assist in re-establishing the balance of the gut microbiota and enhancing gut health by encouraging the development and activity of these advantageous bacteria. Fructooligosaccharides (FOS), galactooligosaccharides (GOS), and inulin are examples of common prebiotics.

Probiotics and prebiotics may work in concert to improve gut health and reduce symptoms of IBS. For those with IBS, this combination—known as synbiotics—can help optimize the advantages of both probiotics and prebiotics.

It's crucial to remember that not all prebiotics and probiotics work the same way and that their effectiveness varies based on the strain, dose, and personal circumstances. Therefore, before beginning any probiotic or prebiotic supplementation plan, particularly if you have IBS or other gastrointestinal issues, it is imperative that you speak with a healthcare provider.

CHAPTER 11

Future Directions And Hope

Advances In Ibs Research

Irritable Bowel Syndrome (IBS) research has been quickly changing in recent years, which gives promise for a better understanding and treatment of this complicated ailment. Understanding the fundamental processes causing IBS is one of the main areas of progress. By exploring the complex interactions among the immune system, neural system, and gut microbiota, researchers are learning more about how these elements affect the onset and course of IBS symptoms.

Furthermore, technological developments have made it possible for scientists to investigate the gut-brain axis in greater depth, providing insight into the reciprocal connection between the stomach and the brain and how it affects symptoms of IBS.

Advanced imaging methods, such as positron emission tomography (PET) scans and functional magnetic resonance imaging (fMRI), have made it possible for researchers to see alterations in brain activity in response to gastrointestinal stimuli, offering important insights into the neurological circuits underlying IBS.

Additionally, several genetic markers linked to an increased risk of IBS have been found via genetic research, providing prospective targets for individualized care. Researchers want to create more specialized treatments that target the unique underlying causes of IBS in each patient by comprehending the genetic base of the illness.

The part that inflammation plays in IBS is another exciting field of study. Although IBS was often thought to be a functional illness, new research indicates that low-grade inflammation may be a major factor in certain IBS symptoms. Anti-inflammatory medicines are now being investigated as possible treatments for certain IBS subtypes as a result of this.

Furthermore, developments in the study of the microbiome have shed light on the intricate connection between gut flora and IBS symptoms. Research has shown that people with IBS have changes in the makeup and functionality of their gut microbiome. These findings suggest that probiotics, prebiotics, and dietary changes may be helpful in modifying gut microbiota and reducing symptoms.

All things considered, these developments in IBS research are encouraging since they may lead to the creation of better diagnostic instruments and therapies that focus on the fundamental causes of the illness, thereby enhancing the lives of those who suffer from IBS.

Promising Therapies On The Horizon

The possible therapy choices for people with Irritable Bowel Syndrome (IBS) are constantly changing along with our knowledge of the ailment. Even though controlling IBS symptoms may be difficult, several exciting new treatments hold promise for better quality of life and symptom management.

Gut-directed hypnotherapy is one new treatment for IBS that has shown encouraging outcomes in clinical studies. To improve symptoms like diarrhea or constipation, bloating, and abdominal discomfort, gut-directed hypnotherapy uses a series of guided relaxation methods and recommendations. Hypnotherapy may assist people with IBS in better managing their symptoms and enhancing their general well-being by addressing the gut-brain link.

Fecal microbiota transplantation (FMT), which entails introducing fecal matter from a healthy donor into the stomach of an IBS patient, is another exciting treatment option. Even while FMT has historically been used to treat recurrent Clostridium difficile infections, a new study indicates that by balancing the gut flora and lowering inflammation, it may also help certain IBS subtypes. At this time, clinical studies are being conducted to assess the safety and effectiveness of FMT for IBS in more detail.

In addition, several cutting-edge pharmaceutical treatments, such as non-absorbable antibiotics, bile acid modulators, and selective serotonin receptor modulators, are being researched for the treatment of IBS. By focusing on certain pathways such as gut microbiota composition, bile acid metabolism, and serotonin transmission that are important in the pathophysiology of IBS, these drugs may provide novel avenues for the treatment of symptoms.

Apart from pharmaceutical and procedural therapy, lifestyle changes continue to be a crucial aspect of managing irritable bowel syndrome. For those with IBS, dietary changes, stress management strategies, and frequent exercise may all help reduce symptoms and enhance overall quality of life.

For those with IBS, the future is bright overall, as more and more treatment choices become available. We may work to provide individuals with IBS greater care and support by expanding our knowledge of the underlying causes of this difficult illness and creating focused therapies.

Living Well With Ibs: Looking Ahead

Although having Irritable Bowel Syndrome (IBS) may come with its own set of difficulties, there are several techniques that people can use to better control their symptoms and enhance their quality of life. In the future, it will be crucial for people with IBS to be proactive about their health and well-being, emphasizing self-care, managing symptoms, and keeping an optimistic mindset.

Living well with IBS requires eating a healthy, well-balanced diet that is customized for each person's requirements and triggers. Maintaining a food journal may assist in pinpointing certain items that worsen symptoms, enabling more focused dietary adjustments. Generally speaking, symptoms may be reduced and gut health can be improved by eating a diet high in fiber, low in FODMAPs (fermentable oligosaccharides, disaccharides, monosaccharides, and polyols), and free of recognized trigger foods like coffee, spicy foods, and artificial sweeteners.

Apart from dietary adjustments, stress reduction methods may be quite helpful in controlling the symptoms of IBS. Many people with IBS have been reported to have worsening gastrointestinal symptoms while under stress, therefore it might be helpful to identify techniques to lower stress levels via mindfulness, meditation, yoga, or deep breathing exercises. Frequent physical exercise may assist regulate bowel function, lower stress levels, and promote overall health and well-being.

In addition, building a supportive medical team is crucial for IBS patients. A general practitioner, gastroenterologist, dietician, or mental health specialist are a few examples of professionals who may provide individualized care and assistance. Being open and honest with medical professionals is essential for creating a personalized treatment plan that takes into account each patient's particular requirements and preferences.

Furthermore, being up to date on the most recent findings and available IBS treatments may enable people to successfully advocate for themselves and make educated healthcare choices. Taking part in online forums or patient support groups may also provide helpful peer support and useful advice for controlling IBS symptoms.

Overall, despite the difficulties this chronic illness presents, people with IBS may live well and flourish by taking a comprehensive approach to treating their disease and proactively addressing symptoms. For those with IBS, there is hope for a better future because of continuous advancements in research and care.

CONCLUSION

In summary, irritable bowel syndrome, or IBS, poses a complicated and diverse challenge to medical professionals as well as patients. A mix of genetic, environmental, and psychological variables contribute to the development of IBS, even if its precise etiology is still unknown. IBS is diverse, which emphasizes the need for individualized treatment plans catered to each patient's requirements.

Considerable progress has been achieved in controlling IBS symptoms and enhancing patients' quality of life, even in the absence of a conclusive treatment. Dietary adjustments, stress reduction strategies, and lifestyle adjustments are essential for symptom control. Furthermore, some people may find relief with medication therapies including antidepressants, laxatives, and antispasmodics.

Furthermore, new studies on the gut-brain axis and the microbiome's function in the pathophysiology of IBS provide hope for the discovery of novel treatment targets. Probiotics, prebiotics, and fecal microbiota transplantation are three current research topics that might change how IBS is managed in the future.

A comprehensive strategy that recognizes the interdependence of social, emotional, and physical elements influencing patients' well-being is necessary for the effective therapy of IBS. Cognitive-behavioral therapy, support groups, and patient education may enable patients to take an active role in their treatment and manage the difficulties that come with IBS.

In summary, even though IBS presents many difficulties, discoveries in the field and improvements in available therapies provide afflicted people hope for improved results.

Collaboration between patients, medical professionals, and researchers may help us improve our knowledge of IBS and create more practical treatment plans for it. Ultimately, managing the complexity of this common gastrointestinal illness requires an all-encompassing and patient-centered strategy.

THE END

www.ingramcontent.com/pod-product-compliance
Lightning Source LLC
Chambersburg PA
CBHW070307230526
45470CB00002B/769